Sugar Cub:

How to Date a Sugar Mama, Cougar, or Rich
Woman

By Brooks Brian

Sugar Cub: How to Date a Sugar Mama, Cougar, or Rich Woman

© 2019 Brooks Brian

Cover by Go On Write at www.goonwrite.com

Disclaimer

This book is about how to have a fulfilling relationship with a woman who is capable of meeting your needs – including your financial needs.

This is not a book about prostitution. It does **not** encourage the reader to break any federal, state, county, city, township, or other local laws.

This book is for entertainment and informational purposes only. It's a relationship advice book. The author is not responsible for anyone acting on any of the ideas and information in this book.

The author is not responsible for any sort of legal damages or any other sort of loss that is claimed to be caused, either in a direct or indirect manner, by any of the entertainment or informational ideas posed in this book.

This book deals with the subject of consenting, healthy, respectful adult relationships. It is written for a mature, 18+ audience.

Please return this book if you don't agree with this disclaimer, or if you are a minor.

Table of Contents

Introduction

Are you tired of forking out hundreds of dollars for dates – with no promise of pleasure at the end?

Wouldn't it be nice if someone else paid for the date? Picked up the check? If someone was actually concerned about your pleasure? If someone took care of your needs, for a change?

Sound too good to be true?

It is - if you date the women around you. You need to reach above and beyond your social circle and your peers. You need to join the secret society of sugar mamas, cougars, and rich women.

In this society, you have a name, a place, and a role.

It's called: sugar cub.

And it may be thing you ever do for yourself.

Forget hanging out with broke girls who expect you to go bankrupt paying for fancy dates. Sit back, relax, and let a rich woman take you to luxurious dinners, fancy resorts, and romantic getaways.

This guide will be short, simple, and easy to understand. My goal is for you to get all the information that you need to immediately go from broke dude to pampered sugar cub.

SECTION 1: Sugar Cub 101

The Benefits of Being a "Kept Man"

Welcome to the wonderful world of sugar cubbing.

In old school terms, this is called being a "kept man." In polite terms, this is a man who financially benefits from his lover. In modern terms, it means a younger man who provides companionship or sex to an older woman. His job is to keep her happy and to be her eye candy.

Think of it as the male equivalent of being a sugar baby.

Why would a man want to date a sugar mama or cougar?

Lots of reasons:
- Gain independence and move out of your parents house
- Pay your rent
- Rising costs of college/help pay your tuition
- Allow you to concentrate on going to school full-time; no need for a job
- Can help you start your own business
- Help you grow your business
- Help you buy a car or fix your car
- Help you buy a motorcycle
- Get out of debt
- Help you pay off a divorce or even child support
- Put away savings
- Start an investment account
- Start a retirement account
- Make a down payment on a home

- Get started in buying investment real estate
- Give you spending money

Inside the Mind of a Rich Woman

Why would a woman want a sugar cub?

The same reason any woman wants to be with a hot man. He's good to look at, he's fun to touch, and he increases her social status and standing, especially amongst her girlfriends.

There are 3 types of women:

1. Single women who are looking for a man
2. Married women who are looking for a man
3. Both married and single women who would be open to having a sugar cub if they found the right man

Although anyone is capable of an affair with a younger man, rich women are especially predisposed to do so. When you already have everything that money can buy, your life becomes boring, predictable. The only thing left to do is age. Having a sugar cub gives an older woman someone to care for and to make her feel young.

However, many women are not honest with themselves about their desires. They would never deliberately go searching for a sugar cub. However, if they found one and that sugar cub made the terms of their relationship clear, they would go for it.

The biggest obstacle you will face as a sugar cub is getting a woman to let down her natural defenses ("I shouldn't" or "He's so young" or "I don't need the trouble of a relationship") long enough to make her see that you will be an improvement to her life, not a detriment.

Don't be afraid to approach a woman and offer to be her sugar cub. The worst she can do is say no – and she'll probably say yes.

Crafting Your Sugar Cub Identity

The first step to becoming a sugar cub is crafting an identity that women will accept, not reject.

You need to make it easy for her to want you as her sugar cub. To do that, you need to show her a man that she will respect and want to help.

That means you need to create an identity that she can respond to with positive feelings and cash.

Below, there are three identities you can choose from. You can mix and match, but you must have at least one of these. That's because if you're not actively studying, working, or starting a business, a woman will think you are a lazy bum. She won't respect you. No respect, no money.

Identity #1: College Student

Women want to help college students. They don't have to feel weird about any cash they give you because they believe it's going to a good cause.

Being a college student is like verbal shorthand for: "I'm going to be a somebody. You should help me to be successful. I'm a future good citizen, who will engage in my community, be a civic leader, volunteer, pay my taxes, buy a home, contribute to the world, etc."

Every time she gives you money, it's practically the same thing as giving to a non-profit. College is understood to be a good thing. You're going to be a better person because you went to college, and she can be a part of that success.

It doesn't even matter what you study. It doesn't matter if you're go to a vocational school, technical school, for-profit school, community college, state school, or university. It doesn't matter if you go part-time or full-time. It doesn't matter if you're traditional college age, or if you're an older student.

Hell, it doesn't even matter if you really go to college or not. You can fake going to college. Go to a thrift store and buy a backpack and some recent looking textbooks. Look up the schedule of your closest college, print out the academic master calendar, and memorize when the semester start and end dates are. Print out a few syllabuses and study guides for some general education classes. Leave them lying around. You get the idea.

Identity #2: Hard Worker Who Just Needs a Leg Up

Women respect men who work hard – even if they're working for minimum wage.

If you can't pull off the college student routine, then be a hard worker.

Work at a low wage job of your choice. It can be something fun and that you love to do. Work for a video game store, a comic book store, work for a clothing store in the mall, work for an automotive shop, work for a motorcycle dealership, work in a bike shop, be a bartender, be a club promoter, work in construction, whatever.

Just work. It doesn't matter where. But you must work.

If you want to work part-time and have your sugar mama supplement your income, fine. But you need to tell her that you work full-time. She'll never know the difference, and she won't be nagging you about why you only work 40 hours a week instead of 20. It's not like she's going to ask to see your paystubs or paycheck deposits.

Women only have sympathy for men who are working hard. She knows you're working retail now, but that you won't be doing it for your whole life.

Women like to improve men. Seeing you bust your ass at a low wage job activates her protective and self-improvement desires. First, she knows that most of your money is going to bills, so she'll be sympathetic to you. She'll want to help you make sure all your bills are paid, and maybe even give you some fun money beyond that. Secondly, she'll want to help you improve your situation in life. If you decide you want to go the college route or the entrepreneur route in order to better your life (or even just pretend like you're going these routes...), she'll open her wallet to help you with that.

Identity #3: Entrepreneur

Women respect men who take action. And when you become an entrepreneur, you're taking action. You're trying to make your life better – and this is something she will bankroll.

If you resent working under someone else's thumb or working for a female boss, your sugar mama can help you to become an entrepreneur.

These are some ideas:
- Start a food truck
- Buy a food franchise
- Become a brewmaster and start selling your own line of beer
- Design apps for smart phones
- Author
- Freelance animator/3D design
- Graphic designer
- Craftsman
- Chef
- Tattoo apprentice
- Website designer
- Webmaster
- Social media consultant
- Product reviewer
- Professional blogger
- E-commerce store owner
- Handyman

One word of caution: most women frown upon video games. So if your idea of entrepreneurship is to becoming a gaming YouTube star, like PewDiePie or ElRubiusOMG or Fernanfloo, don't tell her that. Even if you plan on entering a related field having to do with video games, like game design, game programmer, game script writer, game marketer, or game tech support, she's probably not going to be enthusiastic about it. In fact, you should probably never even tell her you play video games, unless you've heard her express enthusiasm for video games, or she says that she's a gamer herself.

Most women automatically equate gamers with being unmotivated financial leeches with zero ambition. Nothing will make her lose respect for you faster. She may be able to accept that you work in a video game store and that you design video game apps in your spare time, but you should never make it sound like your heart's desire is to work in video games full-time. To her, this will sound like a boy's fantasy – not a man's. Boys don't get respect and money; men do.

SECTION 2: How to Meet Women

Go Where the Women Are

One of the easiest ways to meet women is to come across them in your daily life. So you'll want to get a job where you are likely to encounter lots of women. Particularly single, lonely, wealthy women. You'll also want to consider volunteering and hanging out at places that attract a lot of women.

The three best ways to meet women are using these interests:
1. Home ownership
2. Pets
3. Food

Single women are the single fastest growing segment of home owners. Single women spend, on average, 39.8% of their income on their housing. One of the best ways to meet women is to meet women through housing. Most single women don't start out knowing a lot about home repair.

Most single women are very open to meeting and interacting with men if it related to their home or home improvement.

So, how do you interact with single women and their homes?
- Work at any home improvement store
- Run a handyman business
- Run a lawn care/tree care/snow shoveling/gutter cleaning/chimney cleaning/trash removal/ business
- Install or sell alarm systems

- Install cable
- Install windows, screens
- Paint houses
- Work for a roofing company
- Work for a tree removal service
- Work for a garden center, or the garden section of a major store

Any job that will get you interacting with women in regards to their homes is a win. Most single women outsource any sort of labor related to the home that they can't handle themselves. Wealthy women and career-oriented women are especially likely to outsource this labor.

Another area where you can interact with a lot of single women is through their pets.

Pets have grown in importance over the years, especially as many people are choosing to have pets over children. News articles declare:
- "Fewer Babies, More Pets!"
- "Pets vs. Parenthood: Why More People Are Opting for Pets Over Kids"
- "Fur Babies Over Human Ones"
- "Why I'm Choosing Dogs Over Children"

58% of women own a pet, and many spend lavishly on them.

Getting a job or a hobby that brings you into the orbit of a single, wealthy dog-lover or cat-lover is a natural way to help you connect and start a relationship. Here are some ideas:
- Work at a pet store
- Work as a pet groomer

- Work in a veterinary clinic
- Train dogs
- Housesit pets
- Run a doggy daycare
- Breed dogs or cats
- Professional dog walker
- Work at a feed & tractor store
- Hang out at a dog park
- Build custom hen houses for backyard chicken owners
- Volunteer for an animal rescue
- Volunteer for an animal shelter
- Volunteer at a wildlife sanctuary
- Volunteer at a stable
- Volunteer to raise a Guide Dog for the Blind

The last employment field where you can meet a lot of women is food. Single women spend 11.8% of their income on food – at the supermarket, at the farmer's market, at a specialty stores, etc. They spend 4.4% of their income on eating food outside of the home.

Single women generally won't eat alone at a fancy restaurant, so don't bother getting a wait-staff job in a fine establishment. But they do feel comfortable at casual eateries, like cafes and chain restaurants, coffeeshops and bars. And they also order a lot of takeout.

Here are some food-related jobs that will keep you running into single women:
Pizza delivery driver
- Food delivery drivers (DoorDash, Uber Eats, Food Jets, etc.)
- Counter server at casual eatery
- Bartender

- Barista
- Any position at any coffee shop
- Bagel shop
- Baker/bakery counter/cupcakery/cake or pie or bread store
- Grocery store clerk
- Grocery deliver person

You should also consider spending some of your spare time at places where single women are likely to hang out. Here are some ideas:
- Meditation classes
- Cooking classes
- Yoga studio
- Wellness retreat
- Author event
- Writing workshop
- Bookstore
- Library
- Any store in the mall
- Clothing store
- Wine and beverage store
- Any casual eatery places that are not fast food
- Any kind of coffee or tea shop
- Gym

Finally, another failproof place to meet women is church. The larger, the better. Think: megachurch. There is a well-documented gender imbalance in the churches. Women outnumber men in every Christian denomination. The average American church congregation is 61% female and 39% male.

If you've never been to church or haven't been since you were a child, a megachurch is the best place to start. You can anonymously get lost in the crowd, yet reach out to the church at any time to join a group. Megachurches usually offer dozens of different groups, including mixed gender groups and single groups where you can interact with women. Most of them also have a coffeeshop or a café, a natural place to mingle and strike up conversations with women before or after services.

Approaching Women In Person

Most sugar mamas who you meet in person (i.e. not on a sugar mama dating website) don't think of themselves as sugar mamas. In their minds, they would never have to "pay for it."

Just to be completely clear, your future sugar mama:
- Doesn't think she's a sugar mama
- Would never call herself a sugar mama
- Would be horrified if someone referred to her as a sugar mama
- Doesn't realize you're her sugar cub

Key point: Most sugar mamas don't know that they are sugar mamas.

And you're not going to tell her that she's a sugar mama, either. You're just going to gently guide her behavior into the sugar mama mold, without ever putting a label on what she is.

She's not a sugar mama. She just:
- Helps you out a little
- Helps you with a bill
- Makes sure you have money for food

- Makes up the shortfall in your tuition
- Buys your textbooks
- Makes sure you have something nice every once in a while
- Gifts you a down payment
- Cosigns for you
- Puts you on her cell phone plan/gym membership/Costco card
- Helps you afford your car payment
- Helps you out in an emergency
- Gives you a little something for the holidays
- Buys you lavish gifts for your birthday and Christmas
- Makes sure you're taken care of

Get the idea?

You may be thinking: If it walks like a duck and talks like a duck... - but that's beside the point. Whatever may actually be happening in your sugar mama relationship, you need to just go on pretending that your sugar mama isn't a sugar mama.

Now that you understand that, the question is: how do you approach a woman in person and help her to fit the sugar mama mold?

Start off like you would any other pickup. By making your interest known.

You can't come at a woman with a proposition; you can't come at her demanding thousands of dollars. You approach her and ask her out on a date.

During the date, you will carefully scrutinize the woman to see if she could be a potential sugar mama.

Is this a waste of your time? It could be. But like the old saying goes: you gotta kiss a lot of frogs to get a prince. Or in your case, a rich princess.

Approaching Women Online

Meeting a sugar mama online is much easier than meeting one in person. When you meet one on a sugar mama website, you both know what kind of relationship you're looking for from the start. These are some actual, real-life online advertisements placed by sugar cubs and sugar mamas. (All spelling errors and incorrect punctuation left intact!)

Sugar Cub Ads:

Sugar Cub Ad #1:

I'm looking for a cougar/cub sugar momma kind of relationship. I am 23 years old, 6'4 in shape, fit. I just graduated and would like a nice older woman to spend time with and help me out. Contact me if you want to engage in a mutually beneficial ongoing relationship

Sugar Cub Ad #2:

Hi,

Looking long term sugar mom.

I am 41, look younger. Experienced, educated, entrepreneurial.

Let's get in touch and talk first of all and see if we are can be long term friends

Sugar Cub Ad #3:

I need me a sugar momma to take care of! You looking for a really young man to keep you company? Your house empty and you wanna fill it up a bit? I got you gorgeous ;)!

I am super outgoing, loving, and friendly! I am that person you want around to hang with! I love to do things, we can do anything from go kart racing to skydiving. You name it. Hit me up and lets do things!

Any age welcome, all mommas need loving.

Sugar Cub Ad #4:

I am a college senior looking for a discreet NSA relationship with a mature lady. I am interested in cougars or sugar mommas looking for an athletic, young man. Friends with benefits scenario is also negotiable.

You must be able to host; I cannot host. Prefer someone local--I am willing to meet up at your place. Emphasis on discreet.

Please email reply with a picture of yourself. I can send you pictures of myself after that, and we'll see where it goes. I will only respond to serious inquiries.

Absolutely must be disease-free; this is non-negotiable!

My preferences include Asian females, thick women/BBW, age range 30-52, minimal to no tattoos or piercings. But I'm open-minded to anyone!

I'm handsome, latino, with an athletic build.

Sugar Cub Ad #5:

Hi,

I'm very funny very witty very outgoing very sarcastic easy to get along with don't take life serious always in for a good time

I'm 22 looking for an older woman much older woman to enjoy life together with

Hobbies are cooking gambling playing the piano shopping going on long walks with somebody I could really spend and enjoy time with □

Sugar Cub Ad #6:

I'm 26 fit, smart, funny, and laid back... just looking for someone to take me out and show me a good time.

Sugar Cub Ad #7:

SBM LOOKING FOR COMPANION COUGAR/MILF SUGAR MAMA

Let me know:
1) what you'd like to do?
2) when and where?
3) how frequently
4) how much you can provide?

I offer companionship, body rubs, someone to simply talk to, have drinks, eat, cuddle, etc...

In athletic hwp body shape, 100% ddf, non-smoker with 6 pack, no tattoos, down to earth and a gentleman.
Send your picture and you'll receive mine.

Sugar Mama Ads:

Sugar Mama Ad #1:

Married woman looking for a younger man who can host.

I'll help you out financially.

Sugar Mama Ad #2:

I am looking for a friends-with-benefits situation with a college student who I can help out.

I am educated, professional, and open-minded. I am looking for a college-aged male who needs mentoring and help. Are you struggling financially? I will help you with your bills in exchange for a passionate connection. I have a high sex drive.

Please be drug and disease free. Six pack is a plus.

Sugar Mama Ad #3:

I am a young professional who is too busy to date. I am looking to meet a man my age who needs cash. (I am in my 30's.) I would like to get together once a week.

You must be legitimately single. I have no interest in being the other woman.

Sugar Mama Ad #4:

I am an attorney seeking a WM, unmarried, non-smoking, light social drinker. You must enjoy activities like dinner, going to shows, and working out.

I would like to get together at least 2x/week. I am happy to help you with your rent and other financial needs. This will be part of the terms of an ongoing relationship.

Sugar Mama Ad #5:

I am a wealthy, married WF.

Seeking young man to spoil. I will give you a weekly allowance and a phone that you will use to communicate with me. You need to come when I call. Your allowance will be paid as long as I am happy.

To be considered, you must email me your photos – body and face. Also your allowance requirements or what bills you need help with.

As you can see, there are real men and women out there posting ads and (hopefully!) making good matches.

There are several websites that match sugar cubs with sugar mamas. For example, the website Seeking Arrangement allows sugar cubs and sugar mamas to set up profiles.

You can also look for sugar mamas using regular dating websites. You'll just need to employ certain key words and phrases in your personal ad to let these women know exactly what kind of relationship you're looking for.

In your ad, use any one (or several) of the following terms:
- mutually beneficial relationship
- seeking someone financially generous
- seeking generous lady/woman
- spoil me
- provide companionship
- a good time
- satisfaction guaranteed
- need help with tuition
- need help with bills
- need financial assistance
- seeking allowance
- seeking gifts and other assistance
- seeking woman who is generous to the right man
- seeking cougar
- seeking sugar mama
- wanting to join the sweet life

These key words and phrases should immediately tip a woman off to what kind of relationship you're looking for.

If you're using a regular dating website to attract a sugar mama, make sure you set your age limits high. Like at least from ages 30 to 50. Make it clear that you are open to a woman who is older who can financially support you.

One final word of caution: don't ever send her an unsolicited picture of your cock. Ever. Women receive these photos, unasked for, constantly. It can be upsetting to a conservative, older woman – especially if she opens your message or email at work.

If you must, you send her a picture of your bare midriff. If you do, there better be a 6-pack.

Even if your chat turns sexual, don't send the cock picture. More don't: don't sent a picture of you with your jeans unbuttoned and showing your Happy Trail, don't send a video of you jacking off, don't send a photo of your jizz, and don't send a satisfied and smiling photo of your ex-girlfriend getting a cream pie.

Only send a cock photo if she specifically asks for one. As in: "Please send me a photo of your cock. I want to see it in all of its close up, cut/uncut, vein-popping, discolored glory, preferably held up to a ruler so I can know it's size to the millimeter." Then, and only then, should you send it.

What To Do on the First Date

The first date will show you whether the woman you've selected could be a sugar mama. And more importantly, whether she will be the right sugar mama for you.

On the first date, assuming it's not just coffee, you should pull out all the stops. All the classy gentleman moves. Pull out her chair. Tell the waiter or waitress her order. Compliment her choice. Ask the waiter for a refill on her water, a side of sauce, a napkin, whatever she needs. Listen to her. Ask her lots of questions about herself. Give her flirty little smiles and look in her eyes.

When the bill comes, it's time to make your move. If you do this when the bill comes, it establishes the tone of your relationship – and odds are very, very good that it gets you out of paying the bill.

Do the following:
- Take her hand in yours
- Look into her eyes
- Say: "I don't have much to offer at this stage in my life. I know that I shouldn't, but I feel so strongly about you that I have to ask this question. Do you think you could ever be with a man like me?"

If she asks what you mean by that, simply say: "Poor."

Then wait.

You're not really asking is if she could see herself with a poor man. What you're asking is if she'd be willing to pick up the financial slack in the relationship. If she'd be willing to pay for everything…and to supplement your expenses, as well.

Women are trained to be nice, to be thoughtful. Most of all, they're trained not to be greedy.

Saying that she isn't willing to be with someone who is poor, but who otherwise seems like good person, is taboo. She may think - in private - that she isn't willing to be with someone poor, but admitting it out loud is tantamount to saying you're a terrible person.

No woman wants to admit to being a greedy, selfish, terrible person.

The direct nature of the question will cause her to feel uncomfortable. She won't want to admit to herself how important money is. To protect her own ego and to think of herself as a good person, especially in the face of your bald honesty, she will begin to think:
- "There's more to life than money."
- "He seems like a good person. I'm sure it's not his fault that he's poor."
- "He may be poor now, but he has such potential. He just needs a little help to get there."
- "I'm not so shallow that I would discard a person just because he's poor."

If she responds that she's willing to date you or at least continue communicating with you on some level – as she likely will – then it's time for you to seal the deal. Make a follow up date with her. Ask:
- "When can I see you again?"
- "Would it be alright if I called you?"
- "Could I call you tomorrow?'
- "I'd like to get together again. Maybe next week?"

Let her know that you will be taking the lead in connecting with her. No work required on her part. From now on, your job is to arrange the dates. Her job will be to pay the bills.

And then, follow through. Text or call her the next day. Just tell her you were "thinking of her." Then set up the next date.

Pretty soon, you will be asking for money and then your sugar cub relationship will be paying dividends. But for now, just concentrate on getting her to continue seeing you/dating you.

Now, if she doesn't pick up and pay the bill after your little speech in which you told her you basically couldn't afford to pay, then you still have a few strategies you can deploy.

The first one is to simply ignore the bill. After a few minutes of you not acknowledging the bill, she will grow uncomfortable and restless. Eventually, she will reach for the bill. Smile at her – try to look sheepish – and say nothing.

She should then proceed to pay the bill.

If she still doesn't, smile at her and say: "You know, it's really thoughtful when a woman reverses the gender roles and takes a man out to dinner. Thank you so much."

At this point, she would come across looking like a real bitch by correcting you and making you pay the bill.

If all else fails and she still makes you pay the bill, write it off as a failed sugar cub attempt. She clearly didn't understand what this date was all about. Move on to the next one!

SECTION 3: Make Her Fall For You

Starting the Relationship

So, you went on a first date with your prospective sugar mama. And now you've got a second date lined up.

These initial few dates should be romantic. Assume that she will be paying.

If you're not sure that she's going to pay (she should have gotten the hint by now!) or that she may get cold feet on the second date, then make it a cheap date. This should not be a movie; you want to make a date where she continues to talk about herself. You can't do that if you're sitting in a dark movie theater.

Here are some ideas:
- Indoor or outdoor picnic
- Go for a walk in a park or other pretty surroundings
- Bowling
- Ride bikes (in major cities, you can usually rent bikes)
- Go hiking
- Canoeing, kayaking, or some other outdoor activity
- Cook together
- Go out for ice cream
- Go to a museum
- Go to an art gallery
- Go to a music store
- Go to an open mic night
- Volunteer together

- Do something seasonal – dye Easter eggs, BBQ for the 4th, go on a hayride, go through a corn maze, carve a pumpkin, go look at Christmas lights, go caroling, etc.
- Go on a scenic train ride together, or Amtrak over to the next city
- Take a dance class together
- Take any class together
- Browse a bookstore
- Work on a jigsaw puzzle
- Visit your city's biggest tourist attraction and pretend you're both tourists

On the second date, you should continue to be the charming gentleman who impressed her on the first date. Keep the conversation mostly centered around her.

You should also bring her a very small gift. You already told her you were poor; whatever you give her should reflect that.

In fact, you should give her gifts frequently and throughout the entire relationship.

Why? Shouldn't she be the one giving you gifts?

Yes – and she will. But she's going to feel used or weird if you don't reciprocate. It doesn't matter if she buys you a $500 gift and you reciprocate with a $5 gift. Lovebomb her with small, cheap presents as a way to say: "You're always on my mind."

Here are some ideas:

$0 Ideas:

- Write her a poem
- Hand copy her a romantic poem. Famous poets to choose from: Rumi, Kahlil Gibran, Lord Byron, Shakespeare, Williams Wordsworth
- Memorize a short romantic poem or sonnet and recite it to her
- Burn her a CD of romance music
- Make her a card
- Draw her something
- Pick flowers from an open garden (or a neighbor's yard!)
- Cook for her
- Homemade cookies
- Give her a mix tape, a burned CD, or otherwise personalized playlist
- Write her a love letter

$5 Ideas

- A sappy or romantic card
- Flower: daisies, carnations, or a single rose
- A drink from Starbucks (Bonus points if you know what her favorite is!)
- A "bath bomb" or bubble bath
- Body scrub or sugar scrub
- Gourmet bar of chocolate
- Cute socks
- Cute coffee mug
- A scented candle
- A treat for her pet – cat or dog

$10 Ideas

- Bottle of massage oil
- Buy picnic food. Have an indoor or outdoor picnic

- A teddy bear
- Take her to the movies (matinee)
- Buy a book – most women at least like paperback romance novels
- More elaborate flowers: a small bouquet of roses
- Inexpensive earrings or a piece of jewelry
- Bag of coffee
- Handcrafted soap
- A blank journal and pen

What Women Want in a Lover

What women want in a boyfriend/husband is different than what they want in a lover.

If she were to evaluate you for a long-term relationship, your financial status would be of utmost concern to her. You would fail her test as a permanent prospect.

Fortunately, since you're just being evaluated as a lover/companion and it's known from the beginning that you're the receiver, not bearer, or financial gifts, your sugar mama will evaluate you with by standards that you should easily pass.

These are the kinds of questions that a woman will ask herself while evaluating you:
- Is he good looking?
- Is he mature? Can he carry on a conversation about adult things?
- Will he say or do things out in public that will embarrass me?

- Is he going to talk about other women/past girlfriends?
- Will he answer my texts/calls/email promptly, with lengthy answers and emoticons, or will he treat me like I'm a business associate?
- Does he care if I'm older/overweight/not stylish? Will he treat me like a pity fuck, or will he make me feel like a special, cherished lover?
- If we do make love, will he cum-and-run, or will he spend time afterwards cuddling me?
- If we go shopping/out to dinner/to an event, will he spend the whole time on his phone, looking bored, or make excuses to get away from me? Or will he act like he wants to be there and make me feel like he enjoys spending time with me?

If you've noticed a reoccurring theme in this list, it's that women want to feel special. Even if you're just there for the money, they want to feel like you're her number one priority. Like you'd be with her even if money weren't involved.

So listen to her. Put your phone away and keep it away. Memorize small details about her and reference them at various times in the conversation. Let her talk about what she wants to; ask her lots of questions about herself. For the few hours that you are with her, give her your complete, undivided attention.

Treat it like a job. That's exactly what it is. You are getting paid to make her feel listened to, special, and loved.

SECTION 4: Getting Paid For It

Asking for Money

If you have done everything correctly, your sugar mama should already understand that this is a relationship where you get paid. For the first few dates, she should be signaling her understanding of this arrangement by paying for your dinners. She may already be bringing you gifts.

After the first 2-3 dates, this is the time where you should start asking for money. You have already built a small foundation for your relationship. You have already built an attachment.

You shouldn't let more than three dates elapse before you ask her for money. You don't want her to think she can keep seeing you for free.

Here's how to ask. Ask for a specific amount of money, for a specific purpose. And say please.

Don't promise that it's "just a one time thing" or try to justify asking for money. Just make the request, and wait. Remain silent. She may be silent for several seconds. Wait her out.

- Here are some examples:
  "Could you help me out with $200 for my car insurance bill, please?"
  "I need some help with next semester's textbooks. Could I have $300, please?"
- "There's a rent increase on my apartment and I could use some help. Could I have $100, please?"

- "My car needs repairs. Can I have $400, please?"
- "My next semester of tuition is due. It's $3,400 for the semester. Would you be willing to chip in towards this expense, please? Say, $500?"

Always ask politely.

Make sure that you ask for money for something that is a need, not a want. Cash is for needs. If she asks if she can give you a gift, then it's okay to tell her one of your "wants."

If she's uncomfortable with giving you money, ask her why. Do not ask defensively. Keep your tone curious and polite. She may need to be reassured or have a potential fear allayed before she feels comfortable opening her wallet.

Some of her objections might be:
- "It's too much."
- "I don't know you well enough."
- "I feel like I'm paying you to be with me."
- "I can't afford it."
- "I'm not sure I'm really comfortable with that."

Offer to reduce the amount. If you asked for $500, reduce it to $300. If you asked for $200, reduce it to $100. If you asked for $100, reduce it to $50.

Doing so shows that you don't just view her as an ATM. That it's not all or nothing with you.

It's important that you show flexibility this early in the relationship with how much money you need from her. As she grows more secure in her feelings with the relationship, her generosity will increase. But pushing her or too much, too early on, could scare her and cause her to run.

If she still hesitates, then say:
- "I could really use your help"
- "Your help would really mean a lot to me"
- "It would really make a difference to me"
- "I'm sorry, there's no one else I can ask for help. I just thought maybe we were growing close enough that it was alright for me to turn to you with this problem"

If she refuses entirely or grows visibly uncomfortable, drop the subject. If she apologizes, reassure her that everything is fine. Remain polite and friendly for the duration of your conversation.

Then, once the date is over, don't contact her. Not even so much as a text message. There should be a total wall of silence from your end.

Some women need a few days to think about giving you money.

If you continue to contact her, it shows you're willing to be with her for free.

If you get nasty or demanding with her, you may lose out on a good prospect who just needs a few days to change her mind.

If she contacts you, respond. Keep your response short, but not hostile. Tell her politely that you're busy. No, you don't have time to chat. No, you can't see her right now. Tell her that you're busy working extra hours or that you've taken on a side hustle in order to pay for that bill. Let her think on that for a while. Let her feel a little guilty.

Do not agree to meet with her in person or have any regular contact with her unless she indicates that she is now willing to give you the money.

If she asks you more questions about the bill or why you need money, respond. Offer to show her a copy of the bill.

Many women feel more comfortable paying a bill directly. Meaning, they are willing to write a $600 check to your car insurance company if you show them a physical bill, but they won't hand you $600 directly. Or they'll write a check to your apartment complex office, but they won't give you cash. Or they'll take you to the grocery store and pay for whatever you throw in the shopping cart, but good luck getting the cash otherwise.

Either she'll break down and decide to pay the bill, or she won't. If she doesn't, then you've wasted a little time and a few evenings on a prospect that didn't work out. If she does pay the bill, then you have a sugar mama. Once she's paid one bill, she'll be much more likely to pay the next, and the next, and the next.

Asking for Gifts

A woman who is not comfortable giving you cash will be much more comfortable giving you gifts. This is true even if the gift she's purchasing you costs much more than a cash payment than you initially asked for. For example, she may not be willing to give you $200 in cash, but she is willing to buy you a $1,000 mattress if she discovers you're sleeping on an old futon. Does this make sense? Not really. But it's true!

Women enjoy thinking up gift ideas, shopping for gifts, purchasing gifts, and giving gifts.

The problem is, if you leave the gift giving entirely up to her, she may buy you gifts that you don't need, that aren't practical, that you can't resell, and which take up space and you may resent. She may buy you an incredibly fancy espresso machine that you could care less about, $30 wool socks, matching coffee mugs, a fancy blanket for your couch, a robotic vacuum, whatever.

What you really want is for her to buy you gifts that improve your life, not give you useless clutter.

Gently suggest to her that you would enjoy a different sort of gift. In addition to whatever list you provide her that is tailored to your needs, the following are practical, good suggestions:
- Gift cards to your favorite stores
- Gift cards for gasoline (AM/PM, Chevron)
- Gift cards to grocery stores (Safeway, Albertson's, etc.)
- Gift cards to Amazon
- Prepaid VISA cards
- Textbooks
- Newspaper or magazine subscriptions
- Shopping sprees
- Clothes
- Furniture
- Computer or laptop
- Workout equipment
- Athletic equipment

- Books, CDs, DVDs
- Movie passes
- Memberships, including gym membership, movie club, shaving club, etc.

You can also ask your sugar mama to pay cash for items that are gifts, or for her to pay these expenses directly by paying the bill for the following:
- Security deposit on an apartment
- Down payment on a house
- Car repairs
- Dental work
- Tuition
- Seminar or one-day class on a special subject
- License or certification fees

SECTION 5: Relationship Maintenance

The #1 Mistake That You Must Not Make

The number one mistake you can make in your relationship with your sugar mama is to make her see you as a boy, not a man.

Your behavior, hobbies, and attitude must make her think of you as a man. You must not remind her of her son or her unemployed little brother. Women cannot tolerate a man who sits at home playing video games, smokes pot, sleeps, or goofs off while the other "adults" in the house are working extra hard to keep food on the table and the lights on.

Women must see you as a man in order to respect you. If they don't respect you, they don't want to be with you. Period. Nothing will kill your relationship faster.

Where does this come from?

Maybe she had a negative experience in the past with a boyfriend or an ex-husband who didn't work or barely worked, while she worked full-time and went to school full-time. Maybe he played a ton of video games while she was working two jobs. She didn't feel like he was pulling his weight, and she's still pissed off about it. For her, there's no such thing as water under the bridge!

Or maybe she had a younger brother who was babied by her parents. While she was out in the real world, racking up college degrees, hot-shot internships, and jobs with six-figure starting salaries, Junior was still living at home, smoking pot and working at Taco Time. Maybe she hated the double standard – that she was expected to go out and conquer the world, while her parents made excuses for her baby brother.

Don't do anything that would remind her of a lazy ex-boyfriend or an underachieving little brother.

And as a reminder…you should never, ever talk about your love affair with video games. You shouldn't even tell her that you play video games. You don't need her harping on you about how you choose to spend your spare time.

Other hobbies you should not tell your sugar mama about:
- LARPing and other role-playing games
- Board gaming/tabletop/card games (Cards Against Humanity, Diplomacy, Magic the Gathering)
- Second life gaming
- Cosplay
- Drawing comics or manga
- Comic book collecting
- Watching anime
- Lego building
- Collecting action figures
- Robot combat, competitions
- Building train sets
- Skateboarding
- Smoking pot

So, what's left?

The following is a list of hobbies that your sugar mama will find more acceptable. You probably already do one or more of these:

- Reading (not comic books – almost anything else though, and bonus points if you leave a newspaper lying around)
- Writing
- Intellectual games, like chess or Go
- Traditional card games, like poker
- Anything physical (hiking, kayaking, canoeing, mountain biking, road biking, rafting, rock climbing, rappeling, sailing, scuba diving, skiing, snowboarding, swimming)
- Anything related to playing, not just watching, sports (frisbee, flag football, archery, baseball, basketball, waterskiing, surfing, polo, rugby, fencing, boxing, billiards, volleyball, golf, wrestling, hockey)
- Coaching (Little League, YMCA, Boys & Girls Club, Parks & Rec Center)
- Martial arts (jiu-jitsu, taekwondo, judo, karate, aikido, MMA, etc.)
- Working out (jogging, running, lifting weights, body building, training for a marathon, Ironman, etc.)
- Acting
- Stand-up comedy
- Amateur radio, HAM radio
- Geocaching
- Learning a foreign language
- Anything to do with animals (spending time with your dog, caring for a lizard, exotic fish etc.)
- Homebrewing, beer making
- Photography
- Playing a musical instrument
- Woodworking
- Stock or options trading
- Restoring classic cars

- Motorcycle riding, group riding

Don't get mad if you have to hide certain hobbies from her. Don't get mad if you have to take up a new hobby that you know she will approve of.

She's not your girlfriend. She's your financial sponsor. You don't need to change for her, and you're not going to. You're just going to show her the parts of your personality that will make her respect you and keep her off your back.

Play all the video games you want in private. But when you're with her, talk about your other hobbies.

How to Keep Her Happy

As a sugar cub, you have a specific role in your sugar mama's life.

You bring fun, games, laughter, and good times to her life. To keep her happy, you need to keep things light and fun.

Be wary if your sugar mama seems especially quiet and thoughtful in your presence. Women love to talk – they chatter almost constantly. If she's not talking, she's probably thinking about something deep, and that is a problem for you. Your goal is to bring fun and enjoyment to her life. If she's gone a minute or two without saying anything, ask her "What are you thinking?" Or reach over and squeeze her hand. Or …whatever. Break the spell.

Silence is indicative of a problem. Maybe she's feeling guilty about being with you. Maybe she's reevaluating the relationship. Maybe she's thinking about how little she has in common with you.

Your job is to keep her busy, engaged, and talking. If she's been quiet or moody, suggest that you go out and do a fun activity. Even a walk in the park is better than letting her sit in silence.

Keep her talking, expressing, inquisitive. Keep the conversation going. Your only requirement is to listen and ask the occasional question. Ask her about her feelings, her mood, her thoughts on a particular subject. Then sit back and listen.

SECTION 6: The Party's Over

Ending the Relationship

After a time, either your sugar mama will end the relationship with you, or you will end it with her.

The best kind of endings are the ones where you mutually decide that the relationship isn't working anymore.

She may decide to end the relationship because she met someone else, she can no longer afford you, feels weird about paying you, pressure from family to end the relationship, she moves away, etc.

You may end it because you met someone, you decide that it's no longer worth it, your sugar mama isn't paying you enough, you want to try out a new or different sugar mama, you no longer need the money, or for any other variety of reasons.

My advice is that you save up an emergency fund. This will come in handy if your sugar mama is the one who ends it. Who knows what her timing might be? She might end it right before a big bill is due, or you're about to make a tuition payment. Having an emergency savings account or some kind of cushion will keep you from trying to change her mind, keep you from behaving desperately, or trying to find a new sugar mama in the next 48 hours.

If you're the one who ends it, proceed with caution. Most women handle breakups okay, but every once in a while, a woman can get upset, obsessive, or even stalkerish.

Here are some tips for breaking up with her:

- Don't offer a big explanation about why the relationship is over. If she thinks there's another woman in the picture, it could make her cry or trigger strange, stalkerish behavior
- Tell her simply and firmly that it is time for you to move on
- Tell her you won't be seeing her anymore
- Tell her that you won't be in contact with her, and she shouldn't be in contact with you
- Thank her, sincerely, for all of the help she has given you
- If she begins to cry or get emotional, resist the urge to hug, touch, or kiss her. You don't want her thinking that this behavior will be rewarded with affection; it sets a bad precedent
- No breakup sex

In most cases, your sugar mama will accept your decision and will leave you alone.

If she does become obsessive or weird, then treat her as you would any other stalkerish or psycho ex-girlfriend. This means:

- Don't answer her phone calls
- Don't respond to her messages
- Don't respond to her emails
- Don't accept unwanted gifts
- Don't meet her for sex
- Don't meet her even if she offers you money
- Ignore her if she does a drive-by
- Don't answer her if she comes to your door
- Block her on social media
- Block her phone number
- If you gave her a house key, change the locks

- If she acts suicidal, don't respond to her. Instead, call the police and ask them to do a wellness check at her address

I don't write any of this to scare you. Most sugar mamas are older, mature, and emotionally stable women. It is unlikely that you will need to deal with the above scenario.

Once the relationship is over, you're free to pursue a new sugar mama.

Be a sugar cub for as long as it serves you. You may flit from sugar mama to sugar mama, enjoying years of cash and gifts. Or you may utilize a sugar mama as a one-time only relationship to get you through a rough patch or through college.

Either way, enjoy!

FAQ

Do I need to be a certain age to be a sugar cub?

Yes. You must be at least age 18. No cougar, no matter how daring she is, wants to risk jail time.

That being said, sugar cubs can be of any age. Many women are willing to support a man regardless of age, as long as he makes her happy. Many older men are sugar cubs, but they're completely unaware of it!

Can I have more than one sugar mama at a time?

Yes, though you should never tell your sugar mamas about each other. Women can get very jealous.

Also make sure you manage your schedule in such a way that your sugar mamas never cross paths with each other, or find evidence of one another's existence!

What if I'm not attracted to my sugar mama?

Just pick one thing about her that you think you can deal with, and focus on that.

Also not every sugar cub has sex with his sugar mama. See the next question.

Do I have to have sex with my sugar mama?

No. Many women pay for literally just to have a companion-like relationship. And many women would take a good bubble bath and a massage over sex any day of the week. Draw her a bubble bath, rub her feet, play with her hair, and say something nice. No sex required.

Do I have to buy gifts for my sugar mama?

No, but it will sure improve your odds of keeping your sugar mama happy and generous. A $5 investment here and there can return amazing dividends.

Can I be a sugar cub if I'm overweight or not very handsome?

Yes.

You will discover that a sugar mama's criteria for your appearance is quite possibly much lower than a man's criteria for a woman.

Although it never hurts to look like a male model, sugar mamas keep sugar cubs mostly for how their sugar cub makes them feel, not for the way they look.

Do I need a huge cock?

No. See above. Women care most about how you make them feel, not as much about your body.

Do I need to shave my pubic hair/shave my beard/wax my body/wear special clothes/otherwise change my appearance?

No.

Meet your sugar mama exactly as you are. If she feels strongly about you making changes to your appearance, she will tell you.

Can I get a sugar mama if I have a lot of tattoos and piercings?

Yes.

Some women are very attracted to this look.

However, older conservative women generally are not. If you're meeting an older and/or conservative sugar mama for a first date, consider wearing long sleeves, long pants, and taking any facial piercings out. Over the first date, you should disclose any body art you're hiding. Let her thinking about it without shoving it in her face; she will let you know if it is a deal breaker.

What if she's keeping more than one sugar cub at a time?

That's her right. Just like it is for you to be kept by more than one sugar mama at a time.

What if she wants to take nude photos of me, or film me having sex with her?

Only allow photos/video if you are comfortable with it. Just because she's paying you doesn't mean you have to do everything she says.

Always assume your photos or film could somehow eventually end up on a porn site or otherwise distributed somewhere across the internet. You just never know. If your privacy is important to you, don't allow the photos.

If you do allow photos/video, tell her that you need extra money or gifts for allowing it. You are not an unpaid, amateur porn star. You deserve something extra for it.

What if my sugar mama has stopped giving me money and/or gifts, but still expects to see me?

Except for the initial few dates when you are "building the relationship" you should never see your sugar mama for free. No matter what her excuse is.

Politely tell your sugar mama you'll be happy to see her when she can pay you again. Then stick to your guns. You might be surprised with how quickly she comes up with the money!